I0705775

The Benefits and Risks of Using Organic Apricot Seeds for Cancer Treatment

Wisdom Trail

Copyright © by Wisdom Trail 2024. All right reserved. Before this document is duplicated or reproduced in any manner, the publisher's consent must be gained. Therefore, content within can neither be stored electronically, transferred, nor kept in a database. Neither in part nor full can the document be copied, scanned, faxed, or retained without approval from the publisher or creator

Table of Contents

Chapter 1: Introduction

Overview of Apricot Seeds

Apricot seeds, nestled within the hard shell of the apricot pit, have long been a subject of interest for their potential health benefits. Often overlooked, these small kernels are packed with nutrients and bioactive compounds that have garnered attention in traditional medicine and modern scientific research. Apricot seeds are rich in vitamins, particularly vitamin B17, also known as amygdalin or laetrile, which is at the heart of much of the discussion surrounding their health benefits.

Historically, apricot seeds have been used in various cultures for their supposed medicinal properties. Traditional Chinese medicine, for instance, has utilized apricot seeds for centuries to treat respiratory ailments and other health issues. The seeds are believed to possess anti-inflammatory, antimicrobial, and anticancer properties, making them a focal point in the search for natural remedies.

In recent years, apricot seeds have become a topic of intense debate, particularly concerning their potential role in cancer treatment. Proponents argue that the amygdalin found in apricot seeds can help fight cancer by targeting and destroying cancerous cells. This has led to a surge in interest from individuals seeking alternative or complementary therapies to conventional cancer treatments.

However, the use of apricot seeds is not without controversy. Critics point to the potential risks associated with their consumption, primarily due to the presence of cyanogenic compounds that can release cyanide when metabolized. This has raised safety concerns and led to regulatory scrutiny in various countries. The dichotomy between the perceived benefits and potential dangers has created a complex landscape that requires careful navigation.

Purpose of the Book

The purpose of this book is to provide a comprehensive and balanced exploration of the use of organic apricot seeds in cancer treatment. As interest in natural and holistic health solutions continues to grow, it is crucial to have access to accurate, evidence-based information. This book aims to demystify the claims surrounding apricot seeds, presenting both the potential benefits and the risks associated with their use.

By delving into historical uses, scientific research, and regulatory perspectives, this book seeks to offer a thorough understanding of apricot seeds and their place in modern health discussions. Readers will find an in-depth examination of the nutritional content of apricot seeds, the biochemical mechanisms of amygdalin, and the results of various scientific studies exploring its effects on cancer cells.

Additionally, this book will address the practical aspects of using apricot seeds, including guidelines for safe consumption, potential side effects, and the importance of consulting healthcare professionals before integrating apricot seeds into one's health regimen. The book also differentiates between organic and nonorganic apricot seeds, highlighting the significance of organic farming practices in ensuring product safety and efficacy.

Ultimately, this book aims to empower readers with knowledge, enabling them to make informed decisions about their health. Whether you are exploring apricot seeds as a potential supplement for cancer treatment, or simply curious about their nutritional benefits, this book provides a thorough and objective resource. By the end of this journey, readers will have a well-rounded perspective on apricot seeds, grounded in scientific evidence and mindful of both their promises and pitfalls.

Chapter 2: Understanding Apricot Seeds

Nutritional Profile

Apricot seeds, often referred to as apricot kernels, are a hidden treasure within the fruit, offering a rich array of nutrients and bioactive compounds. These small, almond-like seeds are packed with vitamins, minerals, proteins, and essential fatty acids, making them a notable addition to a balanced diet.

One of the most significant components of apricot seeds is amygdalin, also known as vitamin B17. Amygdalin is a type of cyanogenic glycoside, which means that it can produce cyanide when broken down in the body. This compound is at the center of the debate surrounding the potential health benefits and risks of apricot seeds. Proponents claim that amygdalin has cancer-fighting properties, while critics warn of the toxicity risks associated with cyanide.

Apart from amygdalin, apricot seeds are a good source of protein. They contain around 20-25% protein by weight, providing essential amino acids that are crucial for various bodily functions, including tissue repair and enzyme production. Additionally, they are rich in healthy fats, particularly monounsaturated and polyunsaturated fats, which are known for their benefits to heart health and overall well-being.

Apricot seeds are also abundant in vitamins and minerals. They provide significant amounts of vitamin E, an antioxidant that helps protect cells from oxidative stress and supports skin health. The seeds also contain B vitamins, which play essential roles in energy metabolism and maintaining proper nerve function. Minerals such as magnesium, potassium, and phosphorus are present in apricot seeds, contributing to bone health, muscle function, and electrolyte balance.

Fiber is another important component of apricot seeds, aiding in digestion and promoting a healthy gut. The fiber content helps regulate bowel movements and can contribute to lowering cholesterol levels. Additionally, apricot seeds contain phytosterols, plant compounds that can help reduce cholesterol absorption in the intestines, further supporting cardiovascular health.

Historical and Traditional Uses

The use of apricot seeds dates back centuries, with a rich history rooted in various traditional medicine systems across the globe. In Traditional Chinese Medicine (TCM), apricot seeds, known as "Xing ren," have been used for thousands of years to treat respiratory ailments such as asthma, bronchitis, and coughs. TCM practitioners believe that apricot seeds possess anti-inflammatory and expectorant properties, making them effective in alleviating respiratory symptoms and promoting lung health.

In addition to their use in TCM, apricot seeds have a history in Ayurvedic medicine, the ancient healing system of India. Ayurvedic practitioners have utilized apricot seeds for their purported ability to balance doshas (the body's vital energies) and support overall health. The seeds are believed to have detoxifying properties and are sometimes included in formulations aimed at cleansing the body and improving digestive health.

The Hunza people, an indigenous group residing in the mountainous regions of northern Pakistan, are often cited for their traditional consumption of apricot seeds. The Hunza diet, rich in apricots and their seeds, has been associated with longevity and low incidences of chronic diseases. Some researchers attribute the health and longevity of the Hunza people to their high intake of apricot seeds, although this connection remains a subject of ongoing study and debate.

In the Middle East and parts of the Mediterranean, apricot seeds have been traditionally used for their potential health benefits and as a flavoring agent in various culinary preparations. The seeds are sometimes ground into a paste and added to dishes for their distinct almond-like flavor, and they are also used to make apricot kernel oil, which is valued for its potential health benefits and uses in cosmetics.

Despite their long history of use, apricot seeds have not been without controversy. The presence of amygdalin and its potential to release cyanide has raised safety concerns. In the mid-20th century, amygdalin was extracted and marketed as laetrile, an alternative cancer treatment, sparking considerable debate and regulatory scrutiny. While some early studies suggested potential anticancer benefits, subsequent research and regulatory agencies have highlighted the risks associated with cyanide toxicity, leading to restrictions on the sale and use of laetrile in many countries.

Today, the traditional uses of apricot seeds continue to influence their modern applications, but they are approached with a more critical eye, considering both their historical significance and the findings of contemporary scientific research. As interest in natural and holistic health solutions grows, apricot seeds remain a topic of intrigue, balancing their rich nutritional profile and traditional uses with the need for careful consideration of their potential risks.

Chapter 3: Apricot Seeds and Cancer

Overview of Claims

Apricot seeds have been at the center of a controversial debate regarding their potential role in cancer treatment for decades. Proponents claim that these seeds, particularly their active compound amygdalin (often referred to as vitamin B17), can effectively target and kill cancer cells while sparing healthy tissues. This belief stems from a combination of historical uses, anecdotal reports, and selective interpretations of scientific studies.

The idea that apricot seeds could combat cancer gained significant attention in the 1950s and 1960s when Dr. Ernst T. Krebs Jr., a biochemist, began promoting amygdalin as a natural cancer cure. He coined the term "vitamin B17" to market amygdalin, despite it not being a true vitamin. Krebs and his followers argued that cancer is a deficiency disease, much like scurvy or pellagra, and that supplementing the diet with amygdalin could prevent and treat cancer.

Advocates of apricot seeds and amygdalin as cancer treatments often cite the lower incidences of cancer in populations with high dietary intake of apricot seeds, such as the Hunza people of northern Pakistan. They argue that the seeds' consumption is linked to the health and longevity of these communities, suggesting a protective effect against cancer.

Numerous testimonials and anecdotal reports from individuals who claim to have benefited from apricot seeds also bolster the claims. These personal stories describe significant improvements or complete remissions after using amygdalin, fueling interest and hope among those seeking alternative or complementary cancer therapies.

However, the medical and scientific communities have largely been skeptical of these claims. Critics point out the lack of rigorous clinical evidence supporting the efficacy of amygdalin in cancer treatment and emphasize the potential risks associated with its use. The presence of cyanogenic glycosides in apricot seeds, which can release cyanide, raises significant safety concerns. Regulatory agencies such as the U.S. Food and Drug Administration (FDA) and the European Food Safety Authority (EFSA) have issued warnings and restrictions on the use of amygdalin, citing the dangers of cyanide poisoning.

The Role of Amygdalin and Laetrile

Amygdalin, a naturally occurring compound found in apricot seeds, as well as in the seeds of other fruits like apples, cherries, and peaches, is a cyanogenic glycoside. When metabolized, amygdalin can break down into several components, including hydrogen cyanide, benzaldehyde, and glucose. The release of hydrogen cyanide is central to both the proposed anticancer mechanism and the safety concerns associated with amygdalin.

The mechanism proposed by proponents of amygdalin and laetrile is that cancer cells contain higher levels of the enzyme betaglucosidase, which can hydrolyze amygdalin to release cyanide directly within the tumor environment. The theory suggests that the cyanide selectively targets and kills cancer cells while leaving healthy cells unaffected, as normal cells are believed to have

higher levels of the enzyme rhodanese, which detoxifies cyanide by converting it to thiocyanate, a less harmful compound.

Laetrile, a purified form of amygdalin, was developed to enhance the compound's availability and purported therapeutic effects. Dr. Ernst T. Krebs Jr. and his father, Dr. Ernst T. Krebs Sr., were instrumental in popularizing laetrile as a cancer treatment in the mid-20th century. They claimed that laetrile was more effective and safer than raw apricot seeds, and it was marketed as an injectable or oral supplement.

Despite the compelling theoretical framework and widespread anecdotal support, scientific studies on amygdalin and laetrile have largely failed to demonstrate significant anticancer effects. Early clinical trials conducted in the 1970s and 1980s, including those funded by the National Cancer Institute (NCI), did not show substantial evidence that laetrile was effective in treating cancer. These studies also highlighted the risks of cyanide toxicity, with some patients experiencing adverse effects such as nausea, vomiting, headaches, dizziness, and, in severe cases, cyanide poisoning.

Further biochemical studies have elucidated the pathways through which amygdalin is metabolized. Research published in journals like Cancer Research and Toxicology and Applied Pharmacology has shown that beta-glucosidase, the enzyme that releases cyanide from amygdalin, is not exclusively elevated in cancer cells. Consequently, the potential for cyanide release in healthy tissues raises significant safety concerns.

The metabolic conversion of amygdalin and the associated release of cyanide have led to strict regulations and warnings by health authorities. The FDA has banned the interstate sale and marketing of laetrile for cancer treatment, citing the lack of evidence for its efficacy and the documented risks of cyanide poisoning. Similarly, the EFSA has advised against the consumption of apricot seeds beyond minimal amounts due to the risk of acute cyanide toxicity.

Despite regulatory restrictions, amygdalin and laetrile continue to be used by some alternative medicine practitioners and are available in various forms online and in certain countries. The ongoing debate reflects a broader tension between mainstream medical practice, which prioritizes evidence-based treatments, and alternative approaches that often rely on anecdotal evidence and historical usage.

In summary, while apricot seeds and their active compound amygdalin have been promoted as potential cancer treatments, the scientific evidence to date does not support their efficacy. The risks associated with cyanide toxicity further complicate their use, underscoring the need for caution and rigorous scientific evaluation. The controversy surrounding apricot seeds and cancer treatment illustrates the complexities of integrating traditional remedies into modern medical practice and the critical importance of evidence-based medicine.

Chapter 4: Scientific Research

Studies Supporting Benefits

Scientific interest in apricot seeds, particularly their potential anticancer properties, has spurred numerous studies aimed at understanding their biochemical composition and therapeutic potential. One of the most researched components of apricot seeds is amygdalin, also known as vitamin B17 or laetrile. Proponents of apricot seeds for cancer treatment argue that amygdalin can selectively target and kill cancer cells while leaving healthy cells unharmed.

Several in vitro (test tube) studies have suggested that amygdalin may have anticancer effects. For example, research published in the Journal of Natural Products examined the cytotoxic effects of amygdalin on various cancer cell lines. The study found that amygdalin induced apoptosis (programmed cell death) in cancer cells, particularly in prostate and breast cancer cell lines. The researchers hypothesized that the selective toxicity of amygdalin towards cancer cells could be due to the higher activity of certain enzymes within these cells that convert amygdalin to its active form, releasing cyanide in the process.

Animal studies have also provided some support for the potential anticancer benefits of amygdalin. A study published in Phytotherapy Research investigated the effects of amygdalin on tumor-bearing mice. The results indicated that mice treated with amygdalin exhibited a reduction in tumor size and an increase in survival rates compared to untreated controls. The study suggested that amygdalin might inhibit tumor growth through its proapoptotic effects and its ability to interfere with the metabolism of cancer cells.

In addition to its potential anticancer properties, apricot seeds have been studied for other health benefits. Research has indicated that apricot seeds may have anti-inflammatory and antioxidant effects. A study published in Food Chemistry explored the antioxidant properties of apricot kernel extract and found that it effectively scavenged free radicals and reduced oxidative stress in cells. This antioxidant activity is attributed to the presence of phenolic compounds and vitamin E in the seeds, which can help protect cells from damage caused by oxidative stress.

Another area of interest is the potential cardiovascular benefits of apricot seeds. The monounsaturated and polyunsaturated fatty acids found in apricot seeds are known to support heart health by reducing levels of bad cholesterol (LDL) and increasing levels of good cholesterol (HDL). A study published in the Journal of Agricultural and Food Chemistry demonstrated that apricot kernel oil, rich in these healthy fats, could improve lipid profiles and reduce the risk of cardiovascular disease in animal models.

Studies Highlighting Risks

While the potential benefits of apricot seeds and amygdalin have garnered attention, significant concerns have been raised about their safety. The primary issue is the presence of cyanogenic glycosides, compounds that can release cyanide when metabolized. Cyanide is a potent toxin that can interfere with cellular respiration, leading to symptoms such as headaches, dizziness, confusion, and, in severe cases, death.

Several case reports and clinical studies have documented cyanide poisoning associated with the consumption of apricot seeds. A report published in the British Medical Journal detailed cases of acute cyanide poisoning in individuals who consumed large quantities of apricot seeds. Symptoms include nausea, vomiting, and difficulty breathing, with some cases requiring hospitalization and intensive care.

The potential for cyanide toxicity has led to regulatory scrutiny and restrictions on the sale and use of amygdalin and apricot seeds. The U.S. Food and Drug Administration (FDA) has banned the marketing of laetrile as a cancer treatment due to insufficient evidence of its efficacy and the risks associated with cyanide poisoning. Similarly, the European Food Safety Authority (EFSA) has issued warnings about the consumption of apricot seeds, recommending that adults consume no more than one or two seeds per day to avoid toxic effects.

Further research has examined the metabolic pathways of amygdalin and its conversion to cyanide in the body. A study published in Cancer Research analyzed the enzymatic breakdown of amygdalin and found that the presence of beta-glucosidase enzymes in the intestines and within certain cancer cells can release cyanide. This metabolic process raises concerns about the safety of consuming apricot seeds, particularly in large quantities or without proper guidance.

Moreover, clinical trials investigating the efficacy of laetrile in cancer treatment have largely yielded disappointing results. A comprehensive review published in the Journal of Clinical Oncology evaluated the outcomes of several clinical trials and found no significant evidence that laetrile improved survival rates or reduced tumor size in cancer patients. The review highlighted the risks of cyanide toxicity and recommended against the use of laetrile as a cancer therapy.

Despite the potential health benefits suggested by some studies, the overwhelming evidence of risks associated with cyanide toxicity underscores the need for caution. The scientific community continues to debate the safety and efficacy of apricot seeds and amygdalin, with ongoing research needed to fully understand their potential therapeutic uses and associated dangers.

Chapter 5: Organic vs. Non Organic Apricot Seeds

Differences in Farming Practices

The distinction between organic and non-organic apricot seeds starts with the farming practices employed to cultivate the apricot trees. Organic farming adheres to specific standards and guidelines designed to promote environmental sustainability, biodiversity, and the health of the soil, plants, and ecosystems.

Organic apricot farming prohibits the use of synthetic pesticides, herbicides, and fertilizers. Instead, organic farmers rely on natural methods to manage pests and fertilize crops. This includes the use of compost, manure, green manure, and organic fertilizers to enrich the soil. Natural pest control methods might include introducing beneficial insects, crop rotation, intercropping, and physical barriers to protect the crops from pests.

The avoidance of synthetic chemicals is a cornerstone of organic farming. Organic apricot orchards use biological pest control, such as predatory insects or microbial pesticides, to manage pest populations. Additionally, organic certification standards often require the implementation of soil conservation practices, such as reduced tillage, cover cropping, and the use of organic mulches to maintain soil health and prevent erosion.

Non-organic, or conventional, apricot farming, on the other hand, typically employs a range of synthetic chemicals to manage pests, diseases, and soil fertility. Conventional farmers may use synthetic pesticides and herbicides to protect crops from pests and weeds and chemical fertilizers to enhance soil fertility and boost yields.

These practices can lead to higher productivity and lower costs but may also result in the accumulation of chemical residues on the fruit and in the environment.

Another critical difference lies in the use of genetically modified organisms (GMOs). Organic standards prohibit the use of GMOs in any part of the farming process, from seeds to soil amendments. Conventional farming, however, may utilize GMO seeds designed to resist pests, tolerate herbicides, or improve crop yields.

The certification process for organic farming is stringent. Farms must adhere to organic standards for a minimum period (often three years) before they can be certified as organic. During this transition period, farmers must adopt organic practices but cannot yet label their produce as organic. Regular inspections and audits by certifying bodies ensure that organic farms comply with these standards.

Potential Health Implications

The differences in farming practices between organic and nonorganic apricot seeds can have significant implications for health. One of the primary health benefits associated with organic apricot seeds is the reduced exposure to synthetic pesticides and herbicides. Studies have shown that organic produce generally contains lower levels of pesticide residues compared to conventionally grown produce. Pesticide exposure has been linked to a variety of health issues, including hormone disruption, neurotoxicity, and increased risk of certain cancers.

Organic apricot seeds, therefore, offer a safer alternative for consumers concerned about the potential health risks associated with pesticide residues. The absence of synthetic chemicals in organic farming not only benefits the consumer but also protects farmworkers from exposure to potentially harmful substances. This is particularly important in the context of developing countries, where the use of highly toxic pesticides is more prevalent, and protective measures may be lacking.

Furthermore, organic farming practices that emphasize soil health can enhance the nutritional profile of the produce. Healthy, nutrient-rich soil often leads to crops with higher levels of vitamins, minerals, and antioxidants. Some studies suggest that organic produce may have higher concentrations of certain nutrients, such as vitamin C, iron, magnesium, and phosphorus, as well as phytochemicals that have health-promoting properties.

In the case of apricot seeds, the nutritional differences between organic and non-organic may not be as pronounced as in fruits and vegetables consumed directly. However, the overall health benefits of consuming organic produce, including apricot seeds, extend beyond just nutrient content. The holistic approach of organic farming promotes overall well-being by reducing the intake of harmful chemicals and supporting sustainable agricultural practices.

Another potential health implication of consuming organic apricot seeds is the impact on gut health. Organic farming practices that avoid synthetic chemicals and emphasize biodiversity can support a healthier microbiome in the soil. This biodiversity can translate into a more diverse microbial population on the produce itself, which may benefit the consumer's gut microbiome. A healthy gut microbiome is linked to various health benefits, including improved digestion, enhanced immune function, and reduced inflammation.

Moreover, the environmental benefits of organic farming indirectly support human health. Organic farming practices that reduce pollution, enhance soil fertility, and promote biodiversity contribute to a healthier ecosystem. Clean air, water, and soil are essential for overall public health, and sustainable farming practices play a critical role in maintaining these natural resources.

Conversely, the application of synthetic pesticides and fertilizers in traditional farming practices can result in environmental harm, such as soil degradation, water pollution, and a reduction in biodiversity. These environmental impacts can have far-reaching consequences for human health, as pollutants can enter the food chain and affect communities living near agricultural areas.

While the health benefits of organic apricot seeds are clear, it is essential to recognize that both organic and non-organic apricot seeds contain amygdalin, the compound that can release cyanide. Therefore, regardless of their farming practices, consumers should be aware of the potential risks associated with consuming large quantities of apricot seeds and follow recommended guidelines for safe consumption.

In summary, the choice between organic and non-organic apricot seeds involves considerations of pesticide exposure, nutritional content, environmental sustainability, and overall health impacts. Organic apricot seeds offer a safer and potentially more nutritious option, aligned with principles of environmental stewardship and holistic health.

Chapter 6: Health Benefits

Potential Anti-Cancer Properties

The potential anti-cancer properties of apricot seeds, specifically due to their amygdalin content, have sparked considerable interest and debate. Amygdalin, often referred to as vitamin B17, is a naturally occurring compound found in apricot seeds and other fruit pits. Proponents of apricot seeds for cancer treatment argue that amygdalin can selectively target and kill cancer cells while sparing healthy cells.

The theoretical framework for amygdalin's anti-cancer effects is based on its cyanogenic properties. Amygdalin is a compound that, when broken down, can release cyanide. The proposed mechanism involves the enzyme beta-glucosidase, which is found in higher concentrations in cancer cells than in normal cells. When amygdalin comes into contact with beta-glucosidase, it is hydrolyzed, releasing cyanide directly into the cancerous cells, leading to their destruction. Normal cells, which contain higher levels of the enzyme rhodanese, can detoxify the cyanide, converting it to less harmful compounds like thiocyanate.

Several in vitro studies (test tube experiments) have supported this mechanism. Research published in scientific journals such as the Journal of Natural Products has shown that amygdalin can induce apoptosis (programmed cell death) in various cancer cell lines, including prostate, breast, and colon cancer cells. These studies suggest that amygdalin may inhibit cancer cell proliferation and promote cell death through its cyanogenic action.

Animal studies have also explored the potential anti-cancer effects of amygdalin. For instance, a study published in Phytotherapy Research investigated the effects of amygdalin on tumor-bearing mice. The results indicated that amygdalin treatment led to a reduction in tumor size and an increase in survival rates compared to untreated controls. The researchers proposed that amygdalin's anti-tumor effects might be due to its ability to induce apoptosis and disrupt cancer cell metabolism.

Despite these promising findings, the clinical evidence supporting the use of amygdalin in cancer treatment remains inconclusive and controversial. Several clinical trials conducted in the 1970s and 1980s, including studies funded by the National Cancer Institute (NCI), did not demonstrate significant anti-cancer benefits in humans. These trials also highlighted the risks of cyanide toxicity, with some patients experiencing adverse effects such as nausea, vomiting, dizziness, headaches, and, in severe cases, cyanide poisoning.

Regulatory agencies such as the U.S. Food and Drug Administration (FDA) and the European Food Safety Authority (EFSA) have banned or restricted the use of amygdalin (laetrile) as a cancer treatment due to insufficient evidence of its efficacy and concerns about safety. Despite these restrictions, amygdalin and apricot seeds continue to be used by some alternative medicine practitioners, and anecdotal reports of their benefits persist.

The ongoing debate underscores the need for more rigorous, well designed clinical trials to fully understand the potential anti-cancer properties of apricot seeds and amygdalin. While the theoretical basis and some preclinical studies suggest possible benefits, the lack of consistent clinical evidence and the significant risks associated with cyanide toxicity warrant caution.

Other Health Benefits

Beyond their potential anti-cancer properties, apricot seeds are associated with a variety of other health benefits due to their rich nutritional profile. These seeds are packed with essential nutrients, including vitamins, minerals, proteins, and healthy fats, which contribute to overall health and well-being.

1. Rich Source of Vitamin E:

   Apricot seeds are a good source of vitamin E, a powerful antioxidant that helps protect cells from oxidative stress. Vitamin E is crucial for maintaining healthy skin, eyes, and immune function. It also plays a role in preventing chronic diseases by neutralizing free radicals, which can damage cells and contribute to the development of conditions like heart disease and cancer.

2. Healthy Fats:

   Apricot seeds contain healthy fats, primarily monounsaturated and polyunsaturated fats, which are beneficial for heart health. These fats help lower levels of bad cholesterol (LDL) and increase levels of good cholesterol (HDL), reducing the risk of cardiovascular diseases. The presence of omega-6 and omega-9 fatty acids in apricot seeds supports overall cardiovascular health and helps maintain healthy blood pressure levels.

3. Protein and Amino Acids:

   With approximately 20-25% protein content, apricot seeds provide essential amino acids necessary for various bodily functions, including tissue repair, muscle growth, and enzyme production. Proteins from apricot seeds can be a valuable addition to the diet, especially for individuals looking to increase their protein intake through plant-based sources.

4. Fiber Content:

Apricot seeds are a good source of dietary fiber, which is important for digestive health. Fiber aids in regulating bowel movements, preventing constipation, and promoting a healthy gut microbiome. Additionally, fiber can help lower cholesterol levels and control blood sugar levels, reducing the risk of cardiovascular disease and diabetes.

5. Minerals:

Apricot seeds are rich in essential minerals such as magnesium, potassium, and phosphorus. Potassium helps regulate fluid balance, Magnesium plays an essential role in maintaining proper muscle and nerve function, regulating blood sugar levels, and supporting bone health. Muscle contractions, and nerve signals, while phosphorus is essential for the formation of bones and teeth, DNA synthesis, and energy metabolism.

6. Anti-Inflammatory Properties:

Some studies suggest that apricot seeds may have antiinflammatory effects due to their content of bioactive compounds like phytosterols and polyphenols. These compounds can help reduce inflammation in the body, which is linked to numerous chronic diseases, including arthritis, heart disease, and diabetes.

7. Antioxidant Effects:

The antioxidant properties of apricot seeds, attributed to compounds such as vitamin E, phenolic acids, and flavonoids, help protect the body from oxidative stress and inflammation. Antioxidants play a crucial role in preventing cell damage and reducing the risk of chronic diseases by neutralizing free radicals.

8. Skin Health:

Apricot kernel oil, derived from the seeds, is widely used in skincare products due to its moisturizing and nourishing properties. The oil contains high levels of vitamins A and E, which are advantageous for maintaining healthy skin. It helps maintain skin elasticity, reduces the appearance of fine lines and wrinkles, and protects against UV-induced damage.

While apricot seeds offer a range of health benefits, it is essential to consume them in moderation due to the presence of amygdalin, which can release cyanide when metabolized. Consumers should follow recommended guidelines and consult healthcare professionals before incorporating apricot seeds into their diet, especially in large quantities.

Chapter 7: Risks and Side Effects

Potential Toxicity

The most significant risk associated with apricot seeds is their potential toxicity due to the presence of amygdalin, a cyanogenic glycoside. Amygdalin can release cyanide when metabolized, posing a serious health risk. Cyanide is a potent and fast-acting poison that can interfere with the body's ability to use oxygen, leading to cellular asphyxiation. When consumed in large quantities, apricot seeds can release enough cyanide to cause acute poisoning, which can be fatal.

The toxicity of apricot seeds has led to regulatory scrutiny and warnings from health authorities worldwide. The U.S. Food and Drug Administration (FDA) has banned the marketing of amygdalin (also known as laetrile) as a cancer treatment, citing insufficient evidence of efficacy and the risk of cyanide poisoning. Similarly, the European Food Safety Authority (EFSA) has issued advisories recommending that adults consume no more than one to two apricot seeds per day to avoid toxic effects. For children, even lower amounts are considered safe.

Several factors can influence the cyanide content in apricot seeds, including the variety of apricot, growing conditions, and processing methods. Bitter apricot seeds typically contain higher levels of amygdalin compared to sweet varieties. Therefore, bitter seeds pose a greater risk of cyanide poisoning. Processing methods such as drying, grinding, or cooking can affect the release of cyanide from amygdalin, but they do not eliminate the risk.

Scientific studies have documented cases of cyanide poisoning from apricot seed consumption. Reports published in medical journals highlight instances where individuals experienced acute toxicity after ingesting large amounts of apricot seeds. Symptoms of cyanide poisoning can occur rapidly, often within minutes to a few hours after ingestion, and require immediate medical attention.

The metabolic conversion of amygdalin to cyanide involves several steps. When amygdalin is ingested, it is hydrolyzed by the enzyme beta-glucosidase, which is present in the seeds themselves and the human digestive tract. This hydrolysis releases cyanide, which can then enter the bloodstream. The body's ability to detoxify cyanide is limited, primarily relying on the enzyme rhodanese to convert cyanide to thiocyanate, a less toxic compound. However, the capacity of this detoxification pathway can be overwhelmed by high levels of cyanide, leading to toxic effects.

Symptoms of Overconsumption

Overconsumption of apricot seeds can lead to cyanide poisoning, with symptoms ranging from mild to severe, depending on the amount consumed and the individual's sensitivity to cyanide. Early symptoms of cyanide poisoning may include:

1.   Headache: One of the first signs of cyanide toxicity, caused by the brain's reduced ability to use oxygen.

2.   Dizziness and Confusion: These symptoms result from the central nervous system being affected by low oxygen levels.

3.   Nausea and Vomiting: Gastrointestinal distress is a common response to cyanide ingestion.

4.   Abdominal Pain: This can accompany nausea and vomiting as the digestive system reacts to the toxin.

5.   Weakness and Fatigue: Cyanide interferes with cellular respiration, leading to reduced energy production and general weakness.

6.   Rapid Breathing and Heart Rate: As the body tries to compensate for the reduced oxygen utilization, breathing and heart rate may increase.

As cyanide poisoning progresses, more severe symptoms can develop, including:

7.   Difficulty Breathing: Respiratory distress is a critical symptom, as cyanide prevents cells from utilizing oxygen, leading to a buildup of lactic acid and metabolic acidosis.

8.   Seizures: Severe cyanide poisoning can lead to convulsions as the central nervous system is severely affected.

9.   Loss of Consciousness: In extreme cases, individuals may lose consciousness due to the brain's inability to function without adequate oxygen.

10.   Cardiac Arrest: The heart can be severely affected by cyanide poisoning, potentially leading to cardiac arrest and death if not treated promptly.

Immediate medical intervention is crucial in cases of cyanide poisoning. Treatment typically involves administering antidotes such as hydroxocobalamin, which binds to cyanide and forms a non-toxic compound that can be excreted in the urine. Supportive measures, including oxygen therapy and intravenous fluids, are also essential to manage symptoms and support vital functions.

Chronic exposure to low levels of cyanide, even if not immediately fatal, can have long-term health effects. These may include neurological damage, thyroid dysfunction (due to interference with iodine uptake), and liver and kidney damage. Therefore, even moderate consumption of apricot seeds over an extended period can pose significant health risks.

It is essential for consumers to be aware of the potential dangers associated with apricot seeds and to follow guidelines for safe consumption. This includes adhering to recommended intake limits and being mindful of the type and preparation of the seeds. Pregnant women, children, and individuals with preexisting health conditions should exercise particular caution and consult healthcare professionals before consuming apricot seeds.

In conclusion, while apricot seeds have been promoted for their potential health benefits, the risks associated with their cyanide content cannot be ignored. Understanding the symptoms of overconsumption and the potential toxicity is crucial for safe use. Health authorities continue to advise caution and moderation in the consumption of apricot seeds to prevent serious health consequences.

Chapter 8: Using Apricot Seeds Safely

Recommended Dosages

The consumption of apricot seeds must be approached with caution due to the presence of amygdalin, which can release cyanide when metabolized. Health authorities have provided guidelines on safe intake levels to mitigate the risk of cyanide poisoning.

For adults, it is generally recommended to limit the intake of apricot seeds to a maximum of one to two seeds per day. This conservative recommendation aims to prevent cyanide levels from reaching a toxic threshold. Given the variability in amygdalin content among different apricot varieties and individual seeds, it is prudent to start with a smaller amount and monitor for any adverse effects.

Children are particularly vulnerable to cyanide toxicity due to their smaller body size and lower detoxification capacity. Therefore, children should avoid consuming apricot seeds altogether. If consumption is deemed necessary, it should be strictly limited to small, infrequent amounts, and only under the guidance of a healthcare professional.

Pregnant and breastfeeding women should avoid apricot seeds due to the potential risks posed by cyanide exposure to both the mother and the developing fetus or infant. The toxic effects of cyanide can be particularly harmful during critical periods of development.

Individuals with compromised health, such as those with liver or kidney disease, should also avoid apricot seeds. These organs play a crucial role in detoxifying and excreting cyanide, and any impairment can increase the risk of toxicity.

Despite these recommendations, it is important to note that apricot seeds are not a standardized or regulated product, meaning the amygdalin content can vary widely. Consequently, even adhering to recommended dosages may not guarantee safety in all cases. Consulting with a healthcare provider before incorporating apricot seeds into the diet is essential, especially for individuals with underlying health conditions or those taking medications that may interact with cyanide metabolism.

Preparation and Consumption Tips

Proper preparation and mindful consumption of apricot seeds are essential to minimize the risk of cyanide toxicity. Here are several tips for safely incorporating apricot seeds into your diet:

1. Source and Quality:

Choose high-quality apricot seeds from reputable suppliers who adhere to safety standards. Organic seeds are often preferred to avoid pesticide residues, although organic certification does not impact the cyanide content.

2. Bitter vs. Sweet Seeds:

Be aware of the difference between bitter and sweet apricot seeds. Bitter seeds contain higher levels of amygdalin and are more likely to release dangerous amounts of cyanide. opt for sweet apricot seeds if available, as they have significantly lower amygdalin content.

3. Gradual Introduction:

If you are new to consuming apricot seeds, start with a very small amount, such as half a seed per day, and gradually increase to the recommended dosage. This approach allows you to monitor your body's response and detect any signs of cyanide toxicity early.

4. Grinding and Mixing:

Grinding apricot seeds into a powder can make them easier to incorporate into your diet. However, grinding also increases the surface area, potentially speeding up the release of cyanide. Mix the ground seeds with other foods, such as yogurt, smoothies, or oatmeal, to dilute the concentration and slow down the digestion process.

5. Cooking and Heat Treatment:

While cooking can degrade some of the amygdalin content, it does not eliminate the risk of cyanide release. Heat treatment should not be relied upon as the sole method for reducing toxicity. Instead, combine cooking with other safety measures, such as limiting the quantity consumed.

6. Avoid an Empty Stomach:

Consuming apricot seeds on an empty stomach may increase the absorption rate of cyanide. It is advisable to eat them with meals to slow down digestion and reduce the immediate release of cyanide.

7. Monitor for Symptoms:

Be vigilant for symptoms of cyanide poisoning, especially when first incorporating apricot seeds into your diet. Early signs such as headache, dizziness, nausea, or abdominal pain should prompt immediate cessation of consumption and consultation with a healthcare provider.

8. Storage:

Store apricot seeds in a cool, dry place, away from direct sunlight, to maintain their quality and prevent any potential degradation that might affect amygdalin content.

9. Consult Healthcare Providers:

Always discuss with a healthcare provider before adding apricot seeds to your diet, especially if you have preexisting health conditions, are pregnant or breastfeeding, or are considering giving them to children.

10. Label Reading and Dosage Awareness:

Carefully read product labels for any information on the amygdalin content and recommended dosages. Some products may guide the safe amount to consume based on their specific amygdalin concentration.

Incorporating apricot seeds into your diet requires careful attention to preparation, dosage, and monitoring. By following these guidelines and maintaining open communication with healthcare professionals, you can mitigate the risks associated with their consumption while potentially benefiting from their nutritional properties.

Chapter 9: Legal and Regulatory Considerations

FDA and Other Regulatory Stances

The legal and regulatory landscape surrounding apricot seeds and their derivatives, such as amygdalin (often referred to as laetrile), is complex and varies significantly across different countries and jurisdictions. The U.S. Food and Drug Administration (FDA) and other regulatory bodies worldwide have taken critical stances on these substances due to concerns about their safety and efficacy.

In the United States, the FDA has a clear and firm stance against the use of laetrile as a treatment for cancer. This position is based on extensive evaluations conducted in the 1970s and 1980s, where clinical trials failed to demonstrate any significant anti-cancer efficacy of laetrile. Moreover, these trials highlighted the potential dangers associated with its use, particularly the risk of cyanide poisoning. As a result, the FDA has banned the interstate shipment and marketing of laetrile as a cancer treatment. The FDA's position is supported by major health organizations, including the American Cancer Society and the National Cancer Institute (NCI), both of which have published comprehensive reviews concluding that laetrile is ineffective and dangerous.

The European Food Safety Authority (EFSA) has also expressed concerns about the safety of apricot seeds. In 2016, the EFSA issued a scientific opinion warning that bitter apricot seeds contain high levels of amygdalin, which can release cyanide upon ingestion. The EFSA's risk assessment determined that consuming more than one or two bitter apricot seeds could exceed the safe level of cyanide exposure, particularly for children. Consequently, the EFSA recommends that adults limit their consumption of apricot seeds to a maximum of one to two seeds per day, while children should avoid them altogether. This recommendation is echoed by national food safety authorities across Europe, leading to stringent regulations on the sale and marketing of apricot seeds.

In Canada, Health Canada has issued similar warnings about the potential toxicity of apricot seeds and laetrile. The agency has advised consumers to avoid products containing amygdalin due to the risk of cyanide poisoning. Health Canada also enforces regulations prohibiting the sale of laetrile as a therapeutic product, in line with its mandate to protect public health.

Australia and New Zealand follow comparable regulatory approaches. The Therapeutic Goods Administration (TGA) in Australia has classified laetrile as a prohibited substance due to safety concerns and lack of evidence supporting its therapeutic claims. Likewise, the New Zealand Ministry of Health advises against the use of apricot seeds for medicinal purposes and enforces strict regulations on products containing amygdalin.

Despite these regulatory stances, apricot seeds and amygdalin continue to be available in various forms, often marketed as dietary supplements or natural remedies. This is particularly prevalent online, where vendors can bypass national regulations by selling directly to consumers. As a result, regulatory agencies face ongoing challenges in enforcing their bans and warnings, especially with the global reach of e-commerce platforms.

The regulatory stance against apricot seeds and laetrile is primarily driven by concerns about consumer safety and the lack of credible scientific evidence supporting their use in cancer treatment. Regulatory bodies emphasize the importance of evidence-based medicine and the need to protect consumers from potentially harmful substances that offer no proven benefits.

Legal Status of Laetrile

The legal status of laetrile, the purified form of amygdalin, varies widely across the globe. In the United States, laetrile's legal status has been contentious and subject to extensive legal battles. In the early 1970s, laetrile gained popularity as an alternative cancer treatment, despite the lack of scientific evidence supporting its efficacy. This led to a series of high-profile court cases and regulatory actions.

The FDA's ban on the interstate shipment of laetrile was challenged in court by proponents who argued that patients should have the right to access the treatment. In 1977, a pivotal case, Rutherford v. United States, reached the U.S. Supreme Court. The court ruled in favor of the FDA, upholding its authority to regulate and restrict substances that had not been proven safe and effective. This ruling reinforced the FDA's position and effectively curtailed the legal availability of laetrile within the United States.

Despite the federal ban, some states attempted to pass legislation allowing the use of laetrile within their borders. For example, in the 1970s and 1980s, more than 20 states enacted laws permitting the use of laetrile for terminally ill patients. These state laws, however, were largely symbolic, as the federal ban on interstate commerce of laetrile remained in effect. As a result, access to laetrile in these states was limited and often depended on smuggling the substance from other countries or purchasing it from underground sources.

Internationally, the legal status of laetrile is similarly varied. In Mexico, laetrile is legal and available, often attracting patients from the United States seeking alternative cancer treatments. Clinics in Mexican border towns have long offered laetrile as part of their treatment protocols, marketing it as a natural and holistic option for cancer patients.

In some European countries, laetrile remains illegal due to concerns about safety and efficacy. The European Union's regulations on medical products require rigorous testing and approval processes, which Laetrile has not met. As a result, it is not legally available in the EU, and efforts to market it are met with regulatory enforcement actions.

In contrast, some countries in Asia have a more permissive stance on laetrile. For instance, in parts of Asia where traditional and alternative medicine practices are more integrated into mainstream healthcare, laetrile can be found in certain markets. However, these products often lack regulatory oversight, raising concerns about quality, safety, and the potential for cyanide poisoning.

The legal status of laetrile is influenced by broader debates about the regulation of alternative medicine and the rights of patients to access experimental treatments. Proponents argue that patients, especially those with terminal illnesses, should have the freedom to try alternative therapies when conventional treatments have failed. Critics, however, emphasize the need for rigorous scientific validation and regulatory oversight to protect patients from unproven and potentially harmful treatments.

The ongoing availability of laetrile, despite regulatory bans and warnings, highlights the challenges faced by health authorities in balancing patient autonomy with public safety. It also underscores the importance of continued research and education to ensure that patients and healthcare providers make informed decisions based on credible scientific evidence.

Chapter 10: Consulting Healthcare Professionals

Importance of Medical Guidance

The importance of consulting healthcare professionals before incorporating apricot seeds or their derivatives into your diet or treatment regimen cannot be overstated. Healthcare professionals possess the knowledge and expertise necessary to provide personalized advice based on your health profile, including preexisting conditions, medications, and overall risk factors. Given the potential toxicity of apricot seeds due to their amygdalin content, professional medical guidance is crucial to ensure safety and avoid adverse health outcomes.

Healthcare providers can help assess the risk-benefit ratio of consuming apricot seeds. This is particularly important because the amygdalin in apricot seeds can release cyanide, posing significant health risks if consumed in large quantities. Professionals can offer recommendations on safe dosage, preparation methods, and potential interactions with other treatments or medications. For individuals with specific health conditions, such as liver or kidney disease, healthcare providers can advise on whether apricot seeds are safe to consume and how they might affect the management of their condition.

For cancer patients, consulting healthcare professionals is vital. Apricot seeds have been marketed as a natural cancer treatment, but the scientific evidence supporting their efficacy is limited and controversial. Oncologists and other medical specialists can provide evidence-based advice and discuss the potential risks and benefits of using apricot seeds alongside conventional cancer treatments. They can also monitor for any signs of toxicity and adjust treatment plans accordingly to ensure patient safety.

Pregnant and breastfeeding women should seek medical advice before consuming apricot seeds. The potential risks posed by cyanide exposure to the developing fetus or infant make professional guidance essential. Healthcare providers can offer tailored recommendations to protect both maternal and child health.

Children are particularly vulnerable to cyanide toxicity, and healthcare professionals can guide whether apricot seeds are appropriate for children and, if so, in what quantities. Pediatricians can monitor for any adverse effects and ensure that the child's nutritional needs are met safely.

Moreover, healthcare providers can help interpret and understand the varying regulatory guidelines and warnings issued by health authorities. These guidelines often reflect the latest scientific research and expert consensus on the safety of apricot seeds and related products. By consulting healthcare professionals, individuals can make informed decisions based on the most current and reliable information available.

The role of healthcare professionals extends beyond merely advising on the consumption of apricot seeds. They can also provide a comprehensive approach to health and wellness, considering all aspects of an individual's diet, lifestyle, and medical history. This holistic perspective ensures that any dietary or therapeutic choices, including the use of apricot seeds, are integrated into a broader plan for maintaining or improving health.

Questions to Ask Your Doctor

When discussing the use of apricot seeds with your healthcare provider, it is important to ask detailed and specific questions to ensure you fully understand the potential risks and benefits. Here are some key questions to consider:

1. What Are the Risks of Consuming Apricot Seeds for Someone With My Health Profile?

Ask about the specific risks associated with apricot seeds given your personal health history, including any chronic conditions, allergies, or ongoing treatments. Your doctor can help you understand how these factors may increase the risk of cyanide toxicity or other adverse effects.

2. What Is the Safe Dosage for Apricot Seeds in My Case?

Inquire about the appropriate quantity of apricot seeds that are considered safe for you to consume. This is especially important as the safe dosage can vary widely depending on individual factors such as body weight, age, and overall health.

3. How Should I Prepare and Consume Apricot Seeds to Minimize Risks?

Ask for guidance on the best methods to prepare and consume apricot seeds to reduce the risk of cyanide release. Your doctor may provide tips on grinding, mixing with other foods, or cooking methods that could help mitigate toxicity.

4. Are There Any Signs or Symptoms of Toxicity I Should Watch For?

Understanding the early signs of cyanide poisoning, such as headache, dizziness, nausea, and abdominal pain, can help you identify potential problems early. Ask your doctor to explain what symptoms to look out for and what actions to take if they occur.

5. How Do Apricot Seeds Interact With My Current Medications or Treatments?

Discuss any potential interactions between apricot seeds and your current medications or treatments. Certain medications may affect how your body metabolizes cyanide, increasing the risk of toxicity. Your doctor can advise on any necessary adjustments to your medication regimen.

6. Are Apricot Seeds Safe During Pregnancy or Breastfeeding?

If you are pregnant or breastfeeding, ask specifically about the safety of apricot seeds during these periods. Your doctor can provide advice based on the latest research and guidelines to protect both your health and that of your child.

7. What Alternatives Are Available If Apricot Seeds Are Not Recommended?

If your doctor advises against consuming apricot seeds, inquire about alternative natural remedies or dietary supplements that might offer similar benefits without the associated risks. This can help you find safe and effective options to support your health goals.

8. Can Apricot Seeds Be Part of an Integrative Cancer Treatment Plan?

For cancer patients, ask if and how apricot seeds could be safely integrated into your overall treatment plan. Your oncologist can discuss the potential role of apricot seeds alongside conventional treatments and any necessary monitoring protocols.

9. What Are the Regulatory Guidelines Regarding Apricot Seeds
    in My Region?

Understanding the legal and regulatory status of apricot seeds in
your region can help you make informed choices. Ask your doctor
to explain any relevant regulations and how they impact the
availability and use of apricot seeds.

10. How Often Should I Have Follow-Up Appointments or Tests?

If you decide to incorporate apricot seeds into your diet, discuss
the need for regular follow-up appointments or tests to monitor for
any adverse effects. Your doctor can recommend a schedule for
check-ups and any specific tests that may be necessary to ensure
your safety.

By asking these questions, you can engage in a meaningful
dialogue with your healthcare provider, gaining a comprehensive
understanding of the potential implications of consuming apricot
seeds. This proactive approach helps ensure that any decisions
made are well-informed and aligned with your overall health and
wellness goals.

Summary of Findings

Exploring the use of organic apricot seeds in cancer treatment reveals a complex landscape filled with both intriguing possibilities and significant risks. The seeds, particularly through their content of amygdalin (or vitamin B17), have garnered attention for their purported anticancer properties. Research has shown that amygdalin can induce apoptosis in certain cancer cell lines and reduce tumor growth in animal models. These findings suggest a potential mechanism through which apricot seeds might exert therapeutic effects against cancer, sparking hope among those seeking alternative or complementary cancer treatments.

Moreover, apricot seeds are rich in other beneficial compounds, including healthy fats, proteins, vitamins, minerals, and antioxidants. These nutrients contribute to the overall health benefits of the seeds, supporting cardiovascular health, reducing oxidative stress, and promoting better digestion. The historical use of apricot seeds in traditional medicine systems like Traditional Chinese Medicine and Ayurveda underscores their long-standing reputation as a natural remedy for various ailments.

However, the potential benefits of apricot seeds are significantly overshadowed by the risks associated with cyanide toxicity. Amygdalin, when metabolized, can release cyanide, a potent toxin that poses serious health risks. Numerous case reports and clinical studies have documented instances of cyanide poisoning linked to the consumption of apricot seeds, leading to symptoms ranging from mild discomfort to severe, life-threatening conditions. Regulatory bodies such as the FDA and EFSA have issued warnings and imposed restrictions on the use of apricot seeds and laetrile, emphasizing the dangers of cyanide exposure.

Clinical trials have largely failed to provide robust evidence supporting the efficacy of laetrile as a cancer treatment. Reviews of these trials indicate that laetrile does not significantly improve survival rates or reduce tumor size in cancer patients, further casting doubt on its therapeutic value. The combination of insufficient efficacy data and the clear risks of toxicity has led to a cautious stance within the scientific and medical communities regarding the use of apricot seeds in cancer treatment.

Final Thoughts

The journey through the potential and pitfalls of apricot seeds highlights the importance of a balanced and evidence-based approach to health and wellness. While the allure of natural and holistic remedies is strong, it is crucial to ground our understanding in scientific research and clinical evidence. Apricot seeds, with their rich nutritional profile and historical uses, certainly offer some health benefits, but these must be weighed carefully against the significant risks they pose.

For individuals considering the use of apricot seeds, especially for cancer treatment, it is imperative to consult with healthcare professionals. Medical guidance can help navigate the complexities of potential benefits and dangers, ensuring that any decisions made are informed and safe. The interest in apricot seeds underscores a broader trend toward exploring natural health solutions, but it also serves as a reminder of the need for rigorous research and regulatory oversight to protect public health.

As research continues, it remains essential to approach claims about apricot seeds and similar natural remedies with a critical eye. The scientific community's ongoing efforts to investigate and understand these substances will be key to uncovering their true potential while safeguarding against harm. In the meantime, individuals should prioritize well-established treatments and consult with healthcare providers when considering any new or alternative therapies.

Ultimately, the story of apricot seeds reflects a broader narrative in health and medicine—one of hope, curiosity, caution, and the relentless pursuit of knowledge. By staying informed and seeking professional advice, we can make choices that support our health and well-being safely and effectively.

Your feedback is valuable to us. After reading this book, we invite you to share your thoughts and experiences by leaving a review. Your insights can help others navigate this complex topic and contribute to ongoing discussions about apricot seeds and their potential in health and medicine.

Thank you for embarking on this exploration with us. May your quest for knowledge and wellness be fruitful and enlightening.

www.ingramcontent.com/pod-product-compliance
Lightning Source LLC
Chambersburg PA
CBHW051712250726

48653CB00007B/2993